Alex Esaú Chacón Sevilla

Physical exercise and respiratory therapy Post COVID-19

Alex Esaú Chacón Sevilla

Physical exercise and respiratory therapy Post COVID-19

Physical exercise program for survivors of SARS-CoV-2 induced pneumonia

ScienciaScripts

Imprint

Any brand names and product names mentioned in this book are subject to trademark, brand or patent protection and are trademarks or registered trademarks of their respective holders. The use of brand names, product names, common names, trade names, product descriptions etc. even without a particular marking in this work is in no way to be construed to mean that such names may be regarded as unrestricted in respect of trademark and brand protection legislation and could thus be used by anyone.

Cover image: www.ingimage.com

This book is a translation from the original published under ISBN 978-620-2-25879-1.

Publisher:
Sciencia Scripts
is a trademark of
Dodo Books Indian Ocean Ltd. and OmniScriptum S.R.L publishing group

120 High Road, East Finchley, London, N2 9ED, United Kingdom
Str. Armeneasca 28/1, office 1, Chisinau MD-2012, Republic of Moldova, Europe
Printed at: see last page
ISBN: 978-620-5-64317-4

i.   Summary

This study aimed to determine the effects of a moderate aerobic exercise program combined with respiratory therapy on physical fitness, health-related quality of life, executive functions, and pulmonary function in a survivor of bilateral SARS-CoV-2-induced atypical pneumonia after hospital discharge.

The subject studied was a 35-year-old, single, sedentary man with elementary education who was admitted to the emergency room for 14 days for bilateral atypical pneumonia caused by SARS-CoV-2. The 8-week intervention program consisted of the application of different respiratory exercises plus others aimed at improving cardiorespiratory endurance and muscular strength.

The results show an improvement in physical condition, executive functions, and pulmonary function. However, no evident changes were observed in certain dimensions related to the quality of life expressed by the subject.

It can be concluded, therefore, that this mixed intervention program, based on physical exercise and respiratory therapy, generates positive effects on the physical condition, respiratory function and cognitive capacity of the patient participating in this research.

Key words: pneumonia, physical exercise, respiratory therapy, SARS-CoV-2, physical fitness, executive functions.

ii. Abstract

This study aimed to determine the effects of a moderate aerobic exercise program combined with respiratory therapy on physical condition, health-related quality of life, executive functions, and lung function in a SARS-induced bilateral atypical pneumonia survivor. CoV-2, after discharge from hospital.

The subject studied is a 35-year-old man, single, sedentary, and with elementary studies, who was admitted to the emergency room for 14 days for a bilateral atypical pneumonia caused by SARS-CoV-2. The 8-week intervention program consisted of the application of different respiratory exercises plus others aimed at improving cardiorespiratory endurance and muscular strength.

The results show an improvement in physical condition, executive functions, and lung function. However, no obvious changes were observed in certain dimensions related to the quality of life expressed by the subject.

Therefore, it can be concluded that this mixed intervention program, based on physical exercise and respiratory therapy, generates positive effects on the physical condition, respiratory function and cognitive capacity of the patient participating in this research.

Key words: pneumonia, physical exercise, respiratory therapy, SARS-CoV-2, physical condition, executive functions.

TABLE OF CONTENTS

Chapter 1

1. Introduction

As reported by the Ministry of Health, Equality and Social Affairs (2021), on December 31, 2019, the Wuhan Municipal Health and Sanitation Commission (Hubei Province, China) reported 27 incidences with cases of pneumonia of unknown origin, with a common manifestation in users of a wholesale seafood, fish and live animal market in that city, including 7 severe cases.

Subsequently, on January 7, 2020, Chinese authorities detected, as the triggering agent of the outbreak, a new type of virus of the Coronaviridae family that has been named severe acute respiratory syndrome-inducing coronavirus-2 (SARS- CoV-2), whose genetic sequence was shared by Chinese agencies a week later.

Consequently, on March 11, 2020, WHO announced the 2019 coronavirus disease (Covid-19) as a global pandemic. From this onset until March 19, 2021, more than 112 million cases had been reported worldwide and more than 3 million cases in Spain.

In this country, of the first 18609 infected cases, 43% were admitted to hospital, while 3.9% required admission to the ICU. Thus, the Spanish Society of Internal Medicine (SEMI) initiated a national registry on risk factors for SARS-CoV-2 induced disease (Artero et al., 2021). The study observed a high percentage of patients with comorbidities (61.4% had a moderate or severe Charlson index, 50.9% had arterial hypertension, 39.7% had dyslipidemia, while about 20% had obesity and diabetes), highlighting that 16.5% of patients had a moderate or severe level of dependence to perform activities of daily living (Barthel index less than 60).

Up to June 30, 2020, and according to the SEMI registry, 142 hospital admissions with suspected SARS-CoV-2 infection (48 cases were PCR negative and 94 positive) had been recorded in the Internal Medicine Service of the Hospital García Orcoyen in Estella, Navarra; among them, 66 cases were diagnosed with COVID-19 pneumonia. Of the latter, 20 were confined to their homes and 4 were transferred to the ICU, of whom 1 died and 3 were discharged after treatment with Tocilizumab and steroids, one of them being selected for this study.

Specifically, the patient was diagnosed with bilateral atypical SARS-CoV-2 pneumonia, being referred to the emergency department on November 19, 2020 and discharged on December 3, 2020.

For this reason, the purpose of this research was to test the effect of the intervention carried out with this patient after hospital discharge, based on a program of moderate aerobic exercise combined with respiratory therapy, and which in turn could, in a modest way, suggest or provide recommendations for future research dedicated to subjects who have undergone an illness similar to the one in this study.

This intervention is one of the most relevant aspects of the present study, since emphasis is placed on the combination of physical exercise and respiratory therapy as a therapeutic method to improve the cognitive capacity, physical condition and health-related quality of life of this type of patient. This circumstance is relevant since, according to the responsible medical staff, patients facing this disease in hospitals usually express severe physical and psychosocial complaints caused by the disease and the treatment, especially by the decrease in cardiorespiratory capacities, muscle strength and executive functions.

2. Theoretical framework

2.1. What is Pneumonia?

According to the World Health Organization (WHO), pneumonia is a type of acute respiratory infection that affects the lungs. At the same time, the Clínica Universidad de Navarra (2019) defines pneumonia as an infection that can be caused by multiple organisms (bacteria, viruses and fungi).

For their part, Martinez et al. (2018), interpret pneumonia as inflammatory damage to the lungs in response to the arrival of viruses or bacteria to the distal airway and parenchyma. Despite the concept being histological and microbiological, in clinical praxis the diagnosis rests on the clinical presentation and the demonstration of a radiological pulmonary infiltrate.

The General Directorate of Social Communication (2019) points out that, in the case of pneumonia patients, these organs are filled with pus and fluid, which makes breathing painful and decreases oxygen absorption. In any case, the so-called Community Acquired Pneumonia (CAP) is the most common and is spread by inhaling viruses and bacteria that act as pathogens.

2.2 . SARS-CoV-2 induced pneumonia.

2.2.1. Etiology.

In December 2019, a cluster of pneumonia cases, caused by a newly identified coronavirus p, occurred in Wuhan, China. On January 12, 2020, WHO initially named this coronavirus as 2019-nCoV. Also, this international body officially named the associated disease as COVID-19, while days later the Coronavirus Study Group (CSG) of the International Committee proposed to name the new coronavirus as SARS-CoV-2 (Guo et al., 2020).

Based on the results of virus genome sequencing and evolutionary analysis, it is suspected that the bat is a natural host of viral origin, and SARS-CoV-2 could be transmitted by the bat through unknown intermediate hosts to infect humans. In addition, SARS-CoV-2 could use angiotensin-converting enzyme 2 (ACE2), the same receptor as SARS-CoV to infect humans (Zhou et al., 2020).

2.2.2. Pathology.

Coronaviruses (CoV) belong to the Coronaviridae group, the order Nidovirales and the genus Coronavirus. They are one of the largest groups of viruses that cause respiratory and gastrointestinal infections. Morphologically, CoVs are enveloped viruses containing single-stranded unsegmented positive-sense single-stranded ribonucleic acid (RNA) viruses. SARS-CoV-2 generally causes respiratory and gastrointestinal disease in both humans and animals. The disease is characterized by a variety of medical signs and symptoms including high fever, chills, cough, and shortness of breath or difficulty breathing. Infected individuals may also exhibit other symptoms such as diarrhea, myalgia, fatigue, expectoration, and hemoptysis (Pal et al., 2020).

Along these lines, Pfeifer (2020) states that, from a pathophysiological point of view, COVID-19 pneumonia is a complex acute lung disease with severe damage to the alveolar epithelium and pulmonary-vascular endothelium, resulting in severe respiratory failure in some individuals.

Finally, a recent study published in the American Heart Association (AHA) assures that COVID-19 is a vascular disease and not a respiratory disease. The research reveals that protein S (glycoprotein) alone can damage the endothelial tissue of the body, which is manifested by altered mitochondrial function and eNOS (endothelial synthase) activity increasing glycolytic processes. Thus, once the vascular endothelium becomes infected by SARS-CoV-2, protein S can damage vascular endothelial cells, resulting in endothelitis (Lei et al., 2021).

2.3. What are the signs and symptoms of COVID-19 pneumonia?

WHO has stated that, in the case of pneumonia caused by SARS-CoV-2, the most common symptoms are fever, fatigue and cough, although some patients may experience aches, nasal congestion, rhinorrhea (noticeable nasal discharge), sore throat and even diarrhea. Problems start out mild and appear gradually (Figure 1).

According to the Ministry of Health, Equality and Social Affairs (2021), the greatest experience with COVID-19 comes from the outbreak in China. In this context, 80% of confirmed cases presented mild to moderate symptoms (including cases of mild pneumonia);

13.8% developed a severe clinical course (dyspnea, tachypnea >30/min, O2 saturation < 93%, PaO2/FiO2 < 300, and/or with pulmonary infiltration of > 50% of radiological fields in 24-48%) and 6.1% suffered a critical course (respiratory failure, septic shock and/or multiorgan failure).

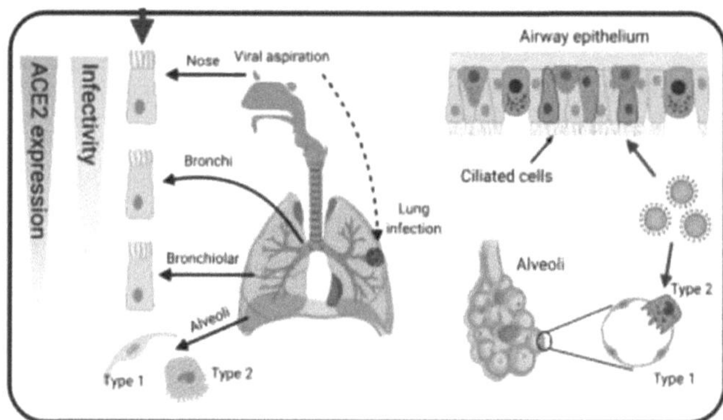

Figure 1. Respiratory system and SARS-CoV-2 infection.

Source: Ministry of Health, Equality and Social Affairs (2021).

2.4. How is Pneumonia diagnosed?

Considering Yurainys et al. (2015) pneumonia can be diagnosed by performing different tests:

- *Sputum test.* It is performed to determine and identify the bacteria that are causing an infection in the lungs or airways.

- *Bronchoscopy.* It is a test used to observe the inside of the airways, being common in the diagnosis of most lung diseases.

- *X-ray.* It is one of the best tests for the diagnosis of pneumonia. Images of the lungs of these patients show white spots called infiltrates, characteristic signs of infection. It can also determine if the patient has any of the complications associated with the disease, such as pleural effusions, i.e. fluid around the lungs.

- CURB-65 Scale. It is an index of the degree of severity for CAP, being useful for predicting a patient's mortality 30 days after diagnosis of pneumonia.

- Blood gas. Measurement of the amount of oxygen and carbon dioxide present in the blood. It is usually accompanied by the determination of blood pH.

2.5. Classification of pneumonia.

In relation to the source of contagion, Alvarez (2016) distinguishes three types of pneumonia: a) community-acquired pneumonia (CAP) or community-acquired pneumonia (CAP); b) nosocomial or hospital-acquired pneumonia (HAP); c) pneumonia associated with the use of mechanical ventilation.

On the other hand, and in reference to the radiological record, pneumonia can be classified according to two syndromes (Dorca et al., 1997). On the one hand, the *typical syndrome,* defined by an acute picture of short duration and characterized by high fever, chills, productive cough and pleuritic chest pain. On the other hand, the *atypical syndrome is* characterized by a more subacute and general type of clinical picture, with fever without chills, headache, myalgia, arthralgia and a particularly troublesome cough lasting several days.

2.6. Treatments for pneumonia.

2.6.1. Pharmacological treatments.

In March 2020, Tocilizumab (TCZ) was included in the seventh diagnostic and treatment plan for SARS-CoV-2 issued by the Chinese health authorities. Similarly, for the treatment of severe pneumonia, in adults with emergency signs (respiratory obstruction or apnea, severe dyspnea, central cyanosis, shock, coma or seizures), airway patency maneuvers are applied and oxygen therapy is administered to achieve blood oxygen saturation (SpO_2) > 94%.

In addition, systemic corticosteroid (SC) therapy is used. However, the therapeutic effects of corticosteroids are often accompanied by clinical side effects, which depend on the dose, route of administration and duration of treatment (Tirapegui and Saldías 2018).

2.6.2. Non-pharmacological therapies.

2.6.2.1. Respiratory therapy.

According to Yurainys et al. (2015), respiratory therapy refers to the set of physical techniques with the aim of removing secretions from the airway and improving lung ventilation. The intervention should be individualized according to the patient's specific needs and conditions.

Recently, Rapela and Capodarco (2021) have carried out a study on pulmonary rehabilitation in a patient with hypoxemia post COVID-19, in which respiratory therapy was based on improving tolerance to physical activity and strengthening of upper and lower limbs, with emphasis on achieving safe walking with the minimum possible assistance. Thus, the authors observed an improvement in the patient's quality of life, and he was able to walk 200 meters without assistance with an oxygen saturation of 93%.

In any case, and in order to generate positive effects, intervention programs based on respiratory therapy should be prolonged for a minimum of 8 weeks (Beauchamp et al., 2011).

2.6.2.2. Exercise-based therapy.

Physical exercise is of great importance and necessity for people who have gone through a serious illness, as it contributes to restore and increase physical condition and quality of life, as has been observed in multiple researches.

In an attempt to establish a certain level of scientific evidence, several studies have been analyzed that confirm the benefits of physical exercise for the improvement of quality of life, physical condition and cognitive capacity in patients with SARS-CoV-2-induced pneumonia.

In their study, Alawna et al. (2021) demonstrated that patients with COVID-19 can safely follow aerobic exercise programs that include 2-3 weekly sessions of 20 to 60 min, performing exercise on a bicycle or simply walking at an intensity of 55% to 80% VO2max or 60% to 80% of maximum heart rate.

Along the same lines, other studies also found positive effects on physical fitness and lung function after the application of combined physical exercise programs with a minimum duration of 6 weeks (Ghodge et al., 2020; Carrasco et al., 2019; Borghi et al., 2009).

2.6.2.3. What are the effects of aerobic exercise on cardiorespiratory fitness and respiratory disease?

Aerobic exercise leads to a greater increase in cardiopulmonary capacity; in addition, it induces immediate improvements in white blood cell action (Mohamed & Alawna, 2020). In a recent systematic review, Gonçalves et al. (2020) have shown that aerobic activities can produce immediate and short-term effects on the immune response of leukocytes, T lymphocytes, lymphocyte subpopulations, interleukins and immunoglobulins. Several authors have shown that a single aerobic exercise session produces improvements in peak immune markers such as T lymphocytes, leukocytes and immunoglobulins.

In this regard, it should be remembered that the activity of the immune system can be significantly affected by the patient's mood. In fact, patients with COVID-19, have a higher tendency to generate anxiety and depression (Huang & Zhao, 2020). Increasing cardiopulmonary capacity can significantly improve mood and thereby improve the capacity of the immune system. This effect could be attributed to the decrease in stress hormones as a consequence of exercise (Nabkasorn et al., 2006).

On the other hand, aerobic exercises can improve the elasticity of lung tissues, increase the strength and endurance of respiratory muscles, improving the recoil mechanism in the respiratory cycle and decreasing the frequency and intensity of cough in case of infection (Mohamed & Alawna, 2020; Borde & Granacher, 2015).

In addition, aerobic exercise plays an antioxidant role in limiting the production of free radicals and so-called oxidative stress (Simioni et al., 2018), while allowing better oxygenation of body and lung tissues (Gagnon et al., 2019). Thus, moderate or mild aerobic exercises can contribute to process these free radicals in the body and prevent the onset of infections and lung diseases such as pneumonia (Artero et al., 2021).

2.7. Functional impact in hospitalized patients with pneumonia. Adequacy of exercise-based therapy.

In patients hospitalized for a serious illness such as pneumonia, among other circumstances, a decrease in physical condition and cognitive function has been observed, which could result in an impairment of their quality of life and their ability to perform their basic daily activities.

As stated by the General Directorate of Public Health and Nutrition (2007) in its physical activity promotion program, it is of vital importance for daily activities to have an excellent cardiopulmonary and/or circulatory capacity that contributes to the correct distribution of oxygen to the body tissues.

In the study by Desai and Needham (2011), a clear increase in mortality was observed in patients who survived the disease but were treated in intensive care units, with impaired pulmonary function being the main cause. In addition, neuromuscular weakness and limitations in both physical fitness and certain aspects of quality of life are common and may be long-lasting.

In this sense, and as indicated by Hoffman (2007), weakness or fatigue of the diaphragm and accessory muscles of inspiration is widely recognized as a consequence of weaning from mechanical ventilation. Fatigue may be due to excessive loading on the inspiratory muscles, which may result from increased airway resistance and/or reduced lung compliance. This same author together with Lj et al. (2015) further note that recovery after sedation is, in most cases, prolonged, with muscle fragility in these patients being a key factor in this regard.

Although, according to Batterham et al. (2014), a high level of evidence has not yet been reached regarding the efficacy of exercise-based interventions in survivors of critical illness after hospital discharge, Paneroni et al., (2021) observed, more specifically, a high prevalence of muscle and physical performance impairment in hospitalized patients without previous locomotor disabilities recovering from COVID-19-induced pneumonia, suggesting the need to implement rehabilitation programs after discharge.

Many recommendations for exercise and physical activity have been published by professional organizations and government agencies since the sui generis publications of the American College of Sports Medicine (ACSM). This body argues that muscular fitness is composed of the functional parameters of strength, endurance and power, each of which improves as a consequence of a properly designed resistance training regimen. As trained muscles become stronger and larger (hypertrophy), endurance must be progressively increased (Table 1) to accumulate additional gains. In any case, it is also necessary to adapt the rest of the variables of this type of training (frequency, volume and rest intervals) to the conditions of the patient in question (ACSM, 1998).

In turn, and as can be seen in Table 4, the American Heart Association (AHA) recommends combining a training program with aerobic exercise and weights. In addition, the WHO proposes 300 minutes of moderate aerobic exercise or also 150 min of vigorous exercise 3 days a week for adults aged 18-64 years, or a combination of both. Likewise, adults should perform muscle-strengthening activity at moderate intensity two or more days a week (WHO, 2020).

On the other hand, the Spanish Association of Cardiology (SEC) and the Spanish Society of Sports Medicine (SEMED), suggest, for subjects confined because of COVID- 19 and/or with chronic diseases, muscle strengthening exercises and aerobic activities (Rodriguez et al., 2020) (Table 2).

Table 1. Aerobic exercise recommendations from the American College of Sports Medicine.

Resumen de recomendaciones preventivas o terapéuticas seleccionadas para actividad aeróbica y los ejercicios de fortalecimiento muscular.

Actividad aeróbica				Actividad de fortalecimiento muscular		
Recomendación	Frecuencia	Intensidad	Duración	Frecuencia	Número de ejercicios	Serie y repeticiones
Enfermedad cardiovascular y la EPOC (2000), American Heart Association (entrenamiento de fuerza y resistencia)	La mayoría, preferiblemente todos los días de la semana	Intensidad moderada a 40 60% del VO_{2max} de reserva (intensidad vigorosa aceptable para adultos seleccionados	30-60 min de actividad de intensidad moderada en episodios de los últimos 10 minutos cada uno	2-3 días a la semana	8-10 ejercicios que involucran los principales grupos musculares	1 serie de 8 a 15 repeticiones (puede progresar a > 1 serie)

Nota: En la tabla solo se proporciona un indicador de intensidad aeróbica, incluso si la recomendación proporciona varios indicadores (comparables). Algunas recomendaciones fueron para actividades de entrenamiento de fuerza, cuando se proporcionó suficiente información en la recomendación, las recomendaciones para la actividad de fortalecimiento muscular se resumieron en forma de un programa de ejercicio que especifica el número de series y el número de repeticiones. Fuente: Adaptado de (Nelson et al., 2007) ACSM, Colegio Americano de Medicina Deportiva; VO_{2max}, capacidad aeróbica máxima.

Table 2. Aerobic and muscle-strengthening exercises for confined subjects during the pandemic.

Resumen de las recomendaciones de las principales instituciones sanitarias sobre el ejercicio

Institución	Aeróbico	Fuerza Muscular
AHA	Ejercicios en circuitos (alternar ejercicios cardiovasculares y de fortalecimiento muscular; 2-3 series cortas cada 30 s) saltos en tijera, saltar a la comba, correr/andar en el mismo sitio, subir escaleras o sobre un step, elevación de piernas, ejercicios de escaladores, saltas en el lugar.	Plancha abdominal y plancha lateral, flexiones, abdominales, levantamiento de caderas o puente, ejercicios de tríceps en una silla, zancada, flexiones ,flexiones isométricas con la espalda apoyada.
COLEF	Pausas activas: caminar por su vivienda, videojuegos activos, rutinas online	Ejercicios de fuerza (propio peso del cuerpo)
SEC/FEC	Pausas activas, andar por la casa, aeróbic, bailar, máquinas para ejercicios cardiovasculares, correr por el salón, avanzar a gatas, saltos laterales	Ejercicios de levantamiento de pesas (p. ej., mancuernas, objetos pesados, paquetes) ejercicios de fuerza con bandas elásticas, flexiones de brazos con una prenda o un cinturón.
SEMED/CGCOM	Pausas activas: caminar por la vivienda, movilizaciones activas.	Ejercicios de levantamiento de pesas (p. ej., mancuernas, botellas, paquetes
OMS	Caminar por la casa, bailar, rutinas de baile online, elevación de piernas a codo, abducciones de piernas, ejercicios aeróbicos, 150 min semanal.	Plancha, abdominal, extensión lumbar, sentadilla, ejercicio de puente lumbar, inmersiones desde silla.

Nota: AHA: American Heart Association; CGCOM: Consejo de Colegios Oficiales Médicos; COLEF: Consejo General de la Educación Física y Deportiva; SEC: Sociedad Española de Cardiología; SEMED: Sociedad Española de Medicina del Deporte; Fuente: Elaboración propia con base en Rodríguez et al. (2020).

In summary, and considering all of the above, the effects generated by SARS-CoV-2 pneumonia, together with hospitalization and treatment to alleviate the sequelae of the disease, will require appropriate intervention in patients who overcome it.

Although, a priori, the approach should be multidisciplinary, the notable affectation that these patients suffer in their physical condition and respiratory function invites to test the effectiveness of a mixed intervention program that, in turn, can generate positive effects on both the cognitive function and the quality of life of these patients.

3. Research problem.

What are the effects of an 8-week moderate aerobic exercise program combined with respiratory therapy on physical fitness, respiratory function, executive functions and health-related quality of life after hospital discharge in a patient with bilateral atypical pneumonia caused by SARS-CoV-2?

Chapter 2

4.   Objectives.

4.1.   General.

To determine the effectiveness of an exercise program combined with respiratory exercises as rehabilitative therapy on physical fitness, respiratory function, executive functions and health-related quality of life in a patient with bilateral atypical pneumonia caused by SARS-CoV-2 after hospital discharge.

4.2.   Specific objectives.

The specific objectives are oriented towards the evaluation of the effects of the mixed intervention program on:

- The muscular strength of the lower limbs and the patient's cardiorespiratory capacity.
- Lung capacity and respiratory functionality.
- Performance on tests designed to examine cognitive impairment and, in particular, the participant's inhibitory control (executive function).
- Health-related quality of life.

5. Methodology.

5.1. Research design.

Single case study.

5.2. Material and methods.

Considering the type of study, the present investigation involved only one surviving patient of bilateral SARS-CoV- 2 induced pneumonia.

On the other hand, and in general, the program, which was preceded by an initial evaluation of the subject, consisted of breathing exercises and a variety of aerobic and muscle strengthening exercises. After 8 weeks from the beginning of the intervention, the patient was re-evaluated under the same conditions that characterized the first evaluation. The study was carried out during the months of January and March 2021, using the patient's own home, as well as the facilities of the Municipal Sports Center of the City of Estella, Navarra.

5.2.1. Description and characteristics of the subject.

Our participant is a 35-year-old man, single, with primary education, unemployed and with previous afflictions (grade II obesity and sleep apnea) (Table 3). In addition, the participant did not engage in any type of physical activity prior to his illness and, for most of the time, was sedentary at home (sitting, watching television or listening to music).

Table 3: Participant description

Características del participante	
Género	Hombre
Edad	35 años
Peso	114.0 kg
Altura	1.76 m
IMC	36.0 Kg/m^2
Nivel Académico	Graduado de primaria
Estado Civil	Soltero
Enfermedades Previas	Apnea del sueño, Obesidad Grado II
Enfermedad Actual	Neumonía SARS-CoV-2

Fuente: Elaboración Propia

On December 1, 2020, the subject was attended at the emergency department of the Hospital de Estella, where he went due to severe dyspnea, and a PCR test for SARS-CoV-2 was performed, which was positive. Likewise, a thoracic A-P X-ray was performed, with a result compatible with bilateral COVID-19-induced pneumonia. Furthermore, the signs and symptoms recorded on admission revealed, in addition to dyspnea, a certain oxygen deficit in the blood, since, although the saturation (SatO2) was slightly above 94%, the respiratory rate was 26-28 cycles per minute.

Once the diagnosis was made, he received treatment with Tocilizumab and several boluses of methylprednisolone, achieving a gradual and progressive improvement until his hospital discharge twelve days later, with a baseline SatO2 of 96%. In any case, given his overweight, he received antithrombotic prophylaxis for thirty days from the date of discharge.

Procedure.

5.2.2.I. Ethical considerations and health safety measures.

This study was carried out in accordance with the principles governing research in humans set out in the Declaration of Helsinki (1964). In this sense, the subject was previously informed of the purpose of the study and of all the actions related to it, emphasizing the confidentiality of the entire process and of the information obtained as a result of their evaluations. Thus, once he had read the corresponding document (appendix), he gave his consent by signing it. Nevertheless, and for reasons beyond the control of the present investigation, it was not possible to complete the report request in the Andalusian Biomedical Research Ethics Portal in due time under the modality of "academic study".

Similarly, the health safety measures proposed by both the WHO and the authorities of Spain and the Autonomous Community of Navarra were taken into account. These consisted basically of the use of masks, hand washing with hydroalcoholic gel or soap and water, disinfection of the instruments or materials used and maintenance of a safe interpersonal distance.)

5.2.2.2. Moderate aerobic exercise program combined with respiratory therapy.

Contents. For the physical exercise program, pedaling on a cycloergometer was used, as well as walking; in addition, for the development of muscular strength, exercises with the patient's own body weight were used (squats, leg push-ups, push-ups on the wall and going up and down stairs at home), exercises with displacement of loads (dumbbells) and exercises with elastic bands. With regard to exercises aimed at improving pulmonary function, an incentive spirometer, balloon inflating and deflating, costal breathing, breathing control techniques, forced exhalation maneuvers such as strong coughing, pursed-lip breathing and diaphragmatic breathing maneuvers were used.

Monitoring-intensity control. With respect to intensity control, the calculation of the reserve heart rate according to Karvonen's formula (HRr) was generally used in each session. In addition, the Borg subjective perception of effort scale (1-10) was applied in order to evaluate the impact generated by each proposed exercise, especially those aimed at developing muscular strength.

In addition to the above, it should be pointed out that, for safety reasons, $SatO_2$ was controlled in each session, avoiding the programmed exercises if the levels of this hematological parameter fell below 94%.

5.2.2.3. Moderate aerobic exercise.

During the first 5 weeks of the intervention, exercise was performed on the cycloergometer and, from the sixth week onwards, outdoor walking on trails was practiced, following the guidelines for aerobic exercise proposed by the WHO, the ACSM, the Spanish Society of Cardiology (SEC), the Spanish Society of Sports Medicine (SEMED) and the AHA.

The aerobic exercises had a frequency of 3 days a week, with a total of 24 sessions (Table 4). During the first 5 weeks, the initial intensity was adjusted between 40-60% of the HR, while, from the sixth week onwards, the intensity was between 60-70% of the HR. In turn, the increase in the duration of the sessions (volume) increased from the sixth week onwards, going from 30 min to 50 min in the final sessions.

Summary of the aerobic exercise program applied in the research.

Programa de Ejercicio Aeróbico

Periodo	Adaptativo	Progreso			
Mesociclo	Inicial	Incremento Progresivo			
Microciclo	Adaptaciones Biológicas	Incremento 1	Incremento 2	Incremento 3	Total
Periodización Lineal	01	01	01	01	01
Semanas	01-05	06	07	08	08
N° de sesiones	15	03	03	03	24
Volumen (min)	30-40	46	50	50	608
Intensidad (%)	40-60	65	70	70	40-70
Series	03	04	04	04	15
Descanso (min)	30	06	06	06	38

Nota. Los ejercicios aeróbicos se realizaron en bicicleta estática más caminatas por senderos de su localidad. Fuente: Elaboración Propia

5.2.2.4. Exercises for the development of muscular strength.

The exercises aimed at developing muscular strength were performed with a frequency of two sessions per week (Table 5). During the first 5 weeks, the subject performed sessions consisting of 2 sets of 8 repetitions using basic exercises (squats, wall push-ups, and biceps curl with dumbbells). From the sixth week onwards, the training sessions were organized as 4 series of 10 repetitions, including, at the same time, new exercises that ensured a harmonious development of strength in both lower and upper body muscles.

Table 5. Physical exercises for muscle strengthening

Ejercicios Fuerza muscular				
Semana	**Ejercicios de Fuerza**	**Ser**	**Rep**	**Descanso**
1-5	Sentadillas, flexiones brazos en la pared, ejercicios de flexiones de brazos con pesas de 5 kg.	2	8	2 min entre serie
6	Subir y bajar escaleras, ejercicios de piernas y brazos con bandas elásticas.	4	10	1 min entre serie
7	Subir y bajar escaleras, ejercicios con bandas elásticas, ejercicios de flexiones de brazos con botellas de agua	4	10	1 min entre serie
8	Subir y bajar escaleras, ejercicios con bandas elásticas, ejercicios de flexiones de brazos con botellas de agua	4	10	1 min entre serie

Nota. Ser. Series Rep. Repeticiones. Antes de la actividad aeróbica se realizaban los ejercicios de fuerza muscular Fuente: Elaboración Propia

5.2.2.5. Respiratory therapy.

As mentioned previously, patients with severe COVID-19 or critically ill patients with respiratory dysfunction should undergo respiratory rehabilitation after discharge.

The exercises developed (Table 6) were selected on the basis of previous studies in which their efficacy had been determined in patients with respiratory failure and/or pneumonia. Thus, the prone position for 2 minutes can aid in dorsal lung ventilation through the reduction of pulmonary compression by the heart due to ventral displacement of the heart (Mccormack, Burnham, & Southern, 2017).

Sitting and standing are the preferred positions in non-critically ill patients to maximize lung function, including forced vital capacity, increase lung compliance and elastic recoil, shift mediastinal structures, and provide a mechanical advantage in forced expiration (Padilla and Muñoz 2017).

Pursed-lip breathing is performed by nasal inspiration followed by expiratory puffing against pursed lips to decrease airway collapse, reduce respiratory rate and dynamic hyperinflation during training with the goal of increasing overall endurance (Wang et al., 2020).

On the other hand, forced expiratory maneuvers such as forceful coughing are indicated to drive secretions (McIlwaine et al., 2017).

According to Wang et al., (2020), pulmonary therapy or activities to improve breathing should be discontinued if $SatO_2$ does not recover and the patient cannot maintain a Borg dyspnea scale score of less than 4 points, with rest and oxygen supplementation recommended. Respiratory rehabilitation exercises should also be discontinued if the patient reports chest pain, palpitations and/or dizziness.

Table 6. Exercise-based respiratory therapy for pulmonary function

Terapia Respiratoria

Semana	Ejercicios para la función pulmonar	Ser	Rep	Descanso
1-5	Ejercicios con labios fruncidos, espiraciones (tos fuerte), respiración diafragmática	8	10	2 min de descanso entre serie
6	Inflar y desinflar globos, espirómetro de incentivo.	4	15	2 min de descanso entre
7	Inflar y desinflar globos, espirómetro de incentivo, respiración costal.	4	15	1 min de descanso entre serie
8	Técnicas de control de la respiración, respiración diafragmática, espirómetro de incentivo.	4	15	1 min de descanso entre serie

Nota. Ser. Series Rep. Repeticiones. Fuente: Elaboración Propia

5.3. Variables.

5.3.1. Respiratory function.

Spirometry is a procedure that facilitates functional evaluation of the lungs in both healthy individuals and patients with respiratory diseases (Yeverino, 2019).

In our study, and taking as a reference the indications of the American Thoracic Society (ATS), forced spirometry was applied using the MIR Spirobank USB spirometer (Rome, Italy). For this, the participant must take in as much air as possible and then abruptly release it until he/she cannot expel any more (Corralo, 2020). It is the most useful for the study of bronchopathies.

According to Graham et al. (2019) the test should be performed in a quiet and comfortable place, with the patient seated (feet should be fully supported on the floor) and upright, keeping the shoulders slightly back and the chin elevated.

The respiratory parameters derived from forced spirometry are shown in Table 7.

Table 7. Relevant parameters derived from forced spirometry

FVC:	Capacidad vital forzada o volumen de aire expulsado mediante una espiración forzada. Se expresa en litros.
FEV₁:	Volumen máximo expulsado en el primer segundo de la espiración forzada. Se expresa en litros.
FEV₁/FVC:	Relación entre FEV₁ y FVC medidos. Puede expresarse en valor absoluto o porcentual (FEV₁%). No debe ser confundido con el índice de Tiffeneau o relación entre FEV₁ y capacidad vital (VC), dado que en circunstancias patológicas la FVC puede ser inferior a la VC debido al colapso dinámico de la vía aérea.
FEF₂₅-₇₅%:	Flujo espiratorio forzado entre el 25% y el 75% de la FVC. Se expresa en litros/segundo.
PEF:	Flujo pico espiratorio o flujo espiratorio máximo conseguido durante la

Fuente: (Javier et al., 2009) disponible en

https://www.neumosur.net/files/consenso_ESPIROMETRIA.pdf

García et al. (2013) argue that the most important variables of forced spirometry are forced vital capacity (FVC) and forced expiratory volume in the first second (FEV₁). FVC reflects the maximum volume of air exhaled in a maximal effort expiratory maneuver, initiated after a maximal inspiration maneuver, expressed in liters. On the other hand, FEV₁ corresponds to the maximum volume of air expelled in the first second of the forced expiratory maneuver, also expressed in liters. In turn, the FEV₁/FVC result shows the relationship between both parameters.

For a correct evaluation of the records obtained in this test, it is necessary to contrast them with certain reference values (Table 8).

Table 8. Normal values within a forced spirometry test

Patrones en función de los datos analizados de la espirometría y sus valores

PATRÓN	FVC	FEV₁	FEV₁/FVC	FEF₂₅₋₇₅ %
Normal	>80 % normal	>80 % normal	>70 % normal	>60 % normal
Obstructivo	>80 % normal	<80 % disminuido	<70 % disminuido	<60 % disminuido
Mixto	<80 % normal	<80 % disminuido	<70 % disminuido	<60 % disminuido
Restrictivo	>80 % normal	>80 % disminuido	>70 % disminuido	<60 % disminuido

Fuente: Elaboración propia, tomado de
https://www.1aria.com/contenido/neumologia/espirometria/neumologia-espirometria-datos-basicos

5.3.2. Physical condition.

5.3.2.I. Cardiorespiratory endurance: 6 min. walking test.

The 6-minute walk test (PC6M) (Rikli and Jones, 1998) allowed us to assess the participant's cardiorespiratory endurance, since, according to Gochicoa et al. (2015), the purpose of such test is to cover, walking as fast as possible, the maximum distance during a period of six minutes.

As indicated above, the $SatO_2$ was monitored during the test in order to avoid any alteration that could worsen the subject's symptom picture. Along the same lines, HR, subjective perception of effort and blood pressure were also recorded.

In relation to the interpretation of the results, the study by Puhan et al. (2008) was taken as a reference, since it concluded that gains of at least 35 m in this test represent significant changes in cardiorespiratory endurance in patients with moderate and severe COPD. On the other hand, the study by Miyamoto et al. (2000) was also considered, who defined a result in this test of 332 m as a cut-off point in terms of survival in patients with primary pulmonary hypertension (below this, survival is 20% at 20 months, while above this survival rate reaches 90%). In this sense, although in probabilistic terms, Lederer et al. (2006), argued that in patients with diffuse pulmonary disease, a 4 times higher mortality is observed in patients who walk less than 207 meters.

5.3.2.2. Test *sit to stand.*

The sit to stand test was applied *to* evaluate the effects of the program on the strength of the patient's lower limb extensor muscles. This test consists of sitting down and getting up from a standard size chair (44 cm high) the greatest number of times (cycles) in 30 seconds. During its development the arms must be crossed and joined to the chest (Vaquero et al., 2015).

As a reference to evaluate the results obtained in the test, the conclusions of the study conducted by Strassmann et al. (2013) were taken, who established that a man aged between 30 and 34 years should perform a minimum of 28 and a maximum of 72 repetitions.

2.3.1. Quality of life.

2.3.1.I. SF-36 questionnaire.

The objective of the SF-36 is to obtain a profile of the perception of health-related quality of life and, given its generic nature, it can be applied to both patients and the general population (Vilagut et al., 2005). In general, people perceive their quality of life according to their personal history, linked to their state of health, prosperity and general well-being (Fleuret & Thouez, 2007).

The original version of the SF-36 is a 36-item scale that assesses 8 dimensions of health: 1) limitations in physical activities due to health problems 2) limitations in social activities due to physical or emotional problems 3) limitations in usual role activities due to physical health problems 4) bodily pain 5) general mental health (psychological distress and well-being) 6) limitations in usual role activities due to emotional problems 7) vitality (energy and fatigue) and 8) general health perceptions. The score obtained in each of these dimensions was set between 0 and 100 points.

5.3.3.2. Sleep quality test (Pittsburgh).

The Pittsburgh Sleep Quality Index (PSQI) is a self-assessed questionnaire designed to assess sleep quality and possible sleep disturbances during the past month. A total of 19 items give rise to seven dimensions or "components": subjective sleep quality, sleep latency, sleep duration, habitual sleep efficiency, sleep disturbances, use of sleep medications and daytime dysfunction. In addition, a global calculation of subjective sleep quality is possible, with a range of scores between 0 and 21 points, where 0 expresses total ease of sleep and 21 maximum difficulty in sleeping considering the seven components (Buysse et al., 1989).

2.3.2. Cognitive Function.

5.3.4.1. Inhibitory control: the stroop effect.

Golden (2005) has demonstrated the usefulness of the color and word test in the assessment of inhibitory control.

Furthermore, this test has been shown in research and practice to be an effective clinical test, both for the assessment of brain dysfunction and for the assessment of psychopathology in general. It can be used as a stand-alone assessment test or as part of a more general battery.

In this case, we used the on-line test available at www.psytoolkit.com, obtaining the number of correct and wrong answers in the three parts of the test (matching words and colors, without semantic interference and with semantic interference).

5.3.4.2. Cognitive impairment: Mini Mental State Examination.

The Mini Mental State Examination (MMSE) consists of a series of questions and tasks whose objective is to evaluate the degree of cognitive impairment present in the person to be evaluated. With the possibility of reaching a maximum score of 30 points, its application does not usually take more than 10 minutes. Its structure includes seven categories, each of which rationally represents a different function: time orientation, place orientation, registration, attention and calculation, spontaneous recall, language (naming, repetition, reading and spontaneous writing) and visual construction (Harvey & Mohs 2001).

5.4 Data analysis.

Being a single case study, the data analysis focused mainly on the pre and post intervention contrast, quantifying the magnitude of the changes both in absolute and relative (percentage) terms.

Chapter 3

6. Results

6.1. Respiratory function.

The intervention program resulted in a very clear improvement in all respiratory parameters evaluated in forced spirometry (PEFVi, FEVi and FVC) (Table 9).

Table 9. Results obtained in forced spirometry.

Forced Spirometry pre- and post-test results

	Pre-Test		**Post-Test**	
Parameters	Pre	Percentage	Post	Percentage
FVC	3.16	73,0	4.38	103,0
FEV1	2.58	71,0	3.66	104,0
PEF	2.87	30,0	8.88	94,0

Note: FVC: forced vital capacity, FEVi: maximum expired volume in the first second, PEF: peak expiratory flow. Source: Own elaboration

6.2. Physical Condition

In the *sit to stand test*, an improvement in lower limb muscle strength was observed, as the patient was able to perform 10 more squats after the intervention was completed (an increase of more than 70%; Figure 2).

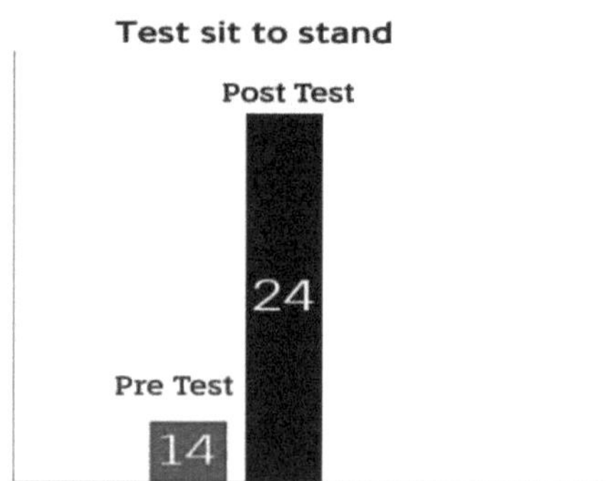

Figure 2. Pre and Post test of the Sit to Stand test. Source: own elaboration.

Figure 3 shows the results obtained in the 6-minute walking test. Taking the previous evaluation as a reference, a clear improvement in cardiorespiratory capacity was observed, as the patient was able to increase the distance covered in the test by 113 meters (23% more). On the other hand, Table 10 reflects the records before and after the test, and in which noticeable changes can be seen in the results related to fatigue, dyspnea, heart rate and blood pressure.

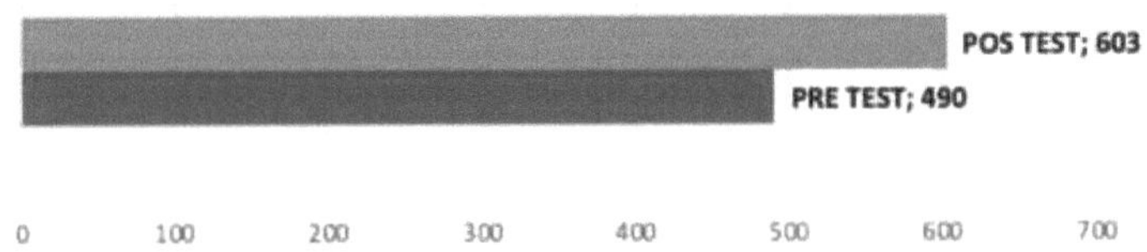

Figure 3. Note: Distance in meters during the pre- and post-test, 6 min walk.

Control of oxygen saturation and heart rate during the pre and post test of the 6 min walk test.

Registro de los signos vitales en la caminata de los 6 minutos					
Tiempo	**FC**	**SpO$_2$**	**Borg disnea**	**Borg fatiga**	**T arterial**
		Pre Test			
Final de prueba	120	95	05	04	130/85
1 minuto	102	96	05	03	130/85
3 minuto	93	98	03	03	125/78
5 minuto	89	98	03	02	127/80
		Post Test			
Final de prueba	110	97	03	03	134/81
1 minuto	93	98	02	02	147/87
3 minuto	92	97	02	01	132/82
5 minuto	90	98	02	01	129/81

Fuente: Elaboración Propia.

6.3 Quality of life and cognitive function.

The data in Table 11 correspond to the results obtained in the SF-36. As can be seen, the intervention program produced a notable increase in the physical (50 points) and emotional (66 points) role-oriented dimensions. Likewise, there was a significant improvement in the pain dimension (23 points). On the other hand, some decreases were observed in the physical and social role scores, as well as in the perception of general health status.

Table 11. Evaluation of health-related quality of life

Calidad de vida (SF 36)	Pre Test	Post Test	Diferencia
Funcionamiento físico	75	65	< 10 P
Limitaciones de roles debido a la salud física	25	75	> 50 P
Limitaciones de roles debido a problemas emocionales	34	100	> 66 P
Energía/Fatiga	65	55	< 10 P
Bienestar emocional	72	68	< 4 P
Funcionamiento social	88	75	< 13 P
Dolor	45	68	> 23 P
Salud general	75	70	< 5 P

Nota. >Mayor <Menor, P puntos Fuente: Elaboración Propia

On the other hand, and considering that, according to the structure of the MMSE, a normal cognitive function can be defined with scores of 24 or more points, the results in this test obtained before the intervention were slightly below this figure (23 points). However, after the intervention, the score on this test reached 27 points, reflecting an improvement in the patient's cognitive status (Table 12).

Similarly, sleep quality improved slightly (Table 12), with a one-point decrease in the score recorded in the pre-intervention assessment.

Table 12. Cognitive function and sleep quality

Prueba	Pre Test	Post Test
Mini Mental	23	27
Calidad de sueño Pittsburgh	07	06

Fuente: Elaboración Propia

In relation to inhibitory control (*stroop* effect*)*, it should be noted that, after the intervention, the patient improved considerably the result of the evaluation performed under semantic interference, notably reducing the number of errors and consequently increasing the number of correct answers while maintaining more or less constant the time spent in responding to the situations presented (Table 13).

Table 13. Inhibitory control before and after the physical exercise program.

El efecto stroop			
Ítems	Color y palabra coinciden	Color sin interferencia semántica	Color con interferencia semántica
		Pre Test	
Fallos	03	00	09
Aciertos	27	30	21
Segundos	303	69	103
		Post Test	
Fallos	06	00	01
Aciertos	24	30	29
Segundos	101	74	104

Fuente: Elaboración Propia

7. Discussion

This single case study, aimed at determining the effects of an exercise program coupled with respiratory therapy of only 8 weeks duration, has generated overall positive effects on physical fitness, respiratory capacity, cognitive function and health-related quality of life in a patient with bilateral pneumonia caused by SARS-CoV-2.

Considering the characteristics of the patient in question, especially his sedentary condition, it was to be expected that the intervention program would generate notable effects on his physical condition. Thus, and taking as a reference the study by Puhan et al. (2008), who established that improvements of 35 meters in the PC6M test represent a minimal detectable improvement in cardiorespiratory capacity in patients with moderate and severe COPD, it can be derived that the increase of 113 meters obtained in this study (almost 25% more compared to the initial evaluation) indicates an important effect of the intervention program in this area. Furthermore, despite this increase in his walking performance, our patient expressed a lower perception of fatigue, as well as an increased ease of breathing during exertion, which reinforces our conclusions in this regard aligning with those obtained by Park et al. (2018).

Regarding muscle strength, the results of the *sit to stand test* after the intervention showed a significant increase (over 70% with respect to the initial evaluation), which practically coincides with the results found by Ghodge et al, (2020) after an 8-week training cut-off similar to that applied in our case; however, according to Strassmann et al. (2013), the performance of a healthy man between 30 and 34 years of age in this test should be, at least, above 28 repetitions or cycles, a figure slightly higher than that finally achieved by our patient at the end of the training period. In spite of this, the effect of the strength exercises included in the program, characterized by being easy to perform and of moderate intensity, managed to provoke muscular adaptations that allow some optimism for the treatment of this type of patient. This is of importance because, as Paneroni et al. (2021) have shown, there is a high prevalence of muscle weakness and impaired physical performance among patients recovering from moderate to severe COVID-19-related pneumonia who were hospitalized without any previous motor limitation.

There seems to be no doubt that exercise-based interventions have a direct effect on respiratory function (Ghodge et al., 2020; Simioni et al., 2018), even improving the symptomatological involvement of pneumonia (Baumann et al. 2012; Borde et al., 2015). If to this is added that the intervention developed in this study contemplated the systematic application of a set of exercises linked to respiratory therapies, it was to be expected that improvements in respiratory function would be evident. In fact, this intervention program managed to reverse the deficits in respiratory function observed in the initial assessment, returning the subject to healthy indices in terms of the three most decisive parameters in forced spirometry: FEVi, PEF and FVC.

As indicated in the introductory section, quality of life can be clearly compromised in patients who develop COVID-19 due to the anxiety produced by the uncertainty of their infection, the poor quality of sleep and the isolation situations that have been required.

The results obtained in our study have pointed to improvements in the importance of the physical and emotional roles of health, although the lack of effects of the program on other dimensions linked to the previous ones makes it difficult to reach more conclusive conclusions in this regard. Furthermore, the changes produced in the quality of sleep after the intervention were minimal, which may have conditioned other more evident changes in the subject's perception of quality of life. In fact, the inverse relationship between treatments, on the one hand, aimed at improving sleep and, on the other, alleviating the respiratory condition of these patients (Liu et al., 2020) could have had an influence not contemplated a priori in this study.

In any case, the results observed here seem to be in line with those previously obtained by Sanjay (2011), who argues that survivors of serious diseases are often left with a legacy of long-term physical, neuropsychiatric and quality of life impairments, to which it should be added that patients with COVID-19 tend to maintain higher degrees of anxiety and depression than other types of patients Huang and Zhao (2020). Finally, with regard to cognitive capacity, significant improvements were observed after the proposed intervention in the patient studied. These results can be considered of great importance because, as has been determined in previous research, patients with chronic hypoxia due to severe pulmonary diseases, such as pneumonia, show a decrease in performance in tests designed to assess attention, processing speed and, in general, executive functions. Like other respiratory viruses, SARS-CoV-2 can enter the CNS through the hematogenous or retrograde neuronal route, producing symptoms such as headache, insomnia, loss of smell and taste which, interestingly, were associated with poor performance in the aforementioned assessment tests (Health et al., 2020; Patricio, 2020).

Apart from the above, and in relation to the limitations of this research, it is necessary to indicate, first of all, that being a single case study, the results obtained in the patient studied after the intervention are subject to multiple conditioning factors that undoubtedly compromise their validity beyond what they imply for the patient studied, and we must be very cautious when extrapolating conclusions to groups with similar or similar ailments.

Another limitation that has influenced the development of the present study has been the interrupted periods of home confinement and personal mobility, which has occasionally made it difficult for the researcher to directly supervise the training sessions.

The lack of economic and material resources has also significantly limited the procedure followed in the study. A more in-depth assessment of the subject by applying hematological and/or imaging tests (e.g., X-ray), as well as the use of appropriate training material and facilities would have enriched the value of this research much more. Nevertheless, we counted on the participation of a physician and a psychologist who not only provided part of the material used here, but also advised the researcher in all aspects related to their professional profiles.

Finally, it is worth mentioning the lack of rigorous studies, either case studies or cohort studies, that would have allowed a more rigorous contrast of the results found here (even hypothesis testing on a mean). The well-known difficulties in counting patients with bilateral pneumonia linked to COVID-19 and also related to safety measures to avoid possible contagion may have reduced the capacity of a good number of researchers in the Physical Activity and Sports Sciences to carry out experimental research to help define the possible evidence on the usefulness of this type of exercise-based therapies.

Chapter 4

8. Conclusions.

Taking into consideration the objectives set out at the beginning of this study, it can be concluded, in view of the results obtained, that the program of physical exercise plus respiratory therapy applied for eight weeks:

- It improved the physical condition of the patient studied, increasing the strength of his leg extensor muscles, as well as his cardiorespiratory capacity.
- The patient's lung capacity and respiratory function clearly improved, resulting not only in higher expiratory values but also in a decrease in exercise-related dyspnea.
- It did not achieve measurable positive effects on all dimensions of health-related quality of life and, moreover, these were minimal on patient-expressed sleep quality.
- It improved, in generic terms, their cognitive function as well as inhibitory control, opening an avenue for the inclusion of exercise-based therapies in the recovery of patients with severe COVID-19-linked pneumonia.

Under these considerations, it can be affirmed, therefore, that the exercise program combined with respiratory exercises as rehabilitative therapy has been effective on physical condition, respiratory function and cognitive functions in a patient with bilateral atypical pneumonia caused by SARS-CoV-2 after hospital discharge.

9. New research perspectives.

In view of the results obtained in the present study, although without forgetting its many limitations, further research should address and test, under experimental designs, the effects of this type of program in patients affected by COVID-19 with bilateral pneumonia and other diseases or comorbidities. At the same time, these experimental studies should examine the effects of these interventions on psychosocial determinants of quality of life.

10. References

Spanish Agency for Medicines and Health Products (2020). Treatments available for the management of SARS-CoV-2 respiratory infection. https://www.aemps.gob.es/la-aemps/ultima-informacion-de-la-aemps-acerca-del-covid-19/tratamientos-disponibles-para-el-management-de-el-manjecion-de-la-inf eccion-respiratoria-por-sars- cov-2/?lang=en

American Psychiatric Association. Diagnostic and Statistical Manual of Mental Disorders. 4th edition. Washington, DC: American Psychiatric Association; 1997.

Aria (2015). Algorithm for the interpretation of a spirometry. https://www.1aria.com/contenido/neumologia/espirometria/neumologia-espirometri a- basic-data

Alawna, m., amro, m., & mohamed, a. a. (2021). Aerobic exercises recommendations and specifications for patients with COVID-19: A systematic review. European Review for Medical and Pharmacological Sciences, 25(24), 13049-13055. https://doi.org/10.26355/eurrev_202012_24211.

Alvarez, J. C. (2016). Pneumonia: Concept, Classification and differential diagnosis. Neumomadrid.org. https://www.neumomadrid.org/wp-content/uploads/monogix_1._neumonias-concept.pdf

Artero, A., Madrazo, M., Fernández-Garcés, M. et al. Severity scores in COVID-19 pneumonia: a retrospective, multicenter, cohort study. *J GEN INTERN MED* 36, 1338-1345 (2021). https://doi.org/10.1007/s11606-021-06626-7.

Aksu, Neriman Temel, Abdullah Erdogan, and Nazmiye Ozgur. 2018. "Effects of Progressive Muscle Relaxation Training on Sleep and Quality of Life in Patients with Pulmonary Resection." Sleep and Breathing 22(3):695-702. doi: 10.1007/s11325-017-1614-2.

Batterham, A. M., Bonner, S., Wright, J., Howell, S. J., Hugill, K., & Danjoux, G. (2014). Effect of supervised aerobic exercise rehabilitation on physical fitness and quality-of-life in survivors of critical illness: An exploratory minimized controlled trial

(PIX study). British Journal of Anaesthesia, 113(1), 130-137.
https://doi.org/10.1093/bja/aeu051.

Baumann, F. T., Zimmer, P., Finkenberg, K., Hallek, M., Bloch, W., & Elter, T. (2012).
Influence of endurance exercise on the risk of pneumonia and fever in leukemia and
lymphoma patients undergoing high dose chemotherapy . A pilot study. December,
638642.

Beauchamp, M. K., Janaudis-Ferreira, T., Goldstein, R. S., & Brooks, D. (2011). Optimal
duration of pulmonary rehabilitation for individuals with chronic obstructive
pulmonary disease - A systematic review. Chronic Respiratory Disease, 8(2), 129-140.
https://doi.org/10.1177/1479972311404256.

Borde, R., Hortobágyi, T., & Granacher, U. (2015). Dose-Response Relationships of
Resistance Training in Healthy Old Adults: A Systematic Review and Meta-Analysis.
Sports Medicine, 45(12), 1693-1720. https://doi.org/10.1007/s40279-015-0385-9.

Borghi-Silva, A., Arena, R., Castello, V., Simões, R. P., Martins, L. E. B., Catai, A. M., &
Costa, D. (2009). Aerobic exercise training improves autonomic nervous control in
patients with COPD. Respiratory Medicine, 103(10), 1503-1510.
https://doi.org/10.1016/j.rmed.2009.04.015.

Buysse, D. J., Reynolds, C. F., Monk, T. H., Berman, S. R., & Kupfer, D. J. (1989). Buysse
DJ, Reynolds CF, Monk TH, Berman SR, Kupfer DJ. The Pittsburgh Sleep Quality
Index: a new instrument for psychiatric practice and research. Psychiatry Res.
1989;28:193-213.

Carrasco Martínez, A. J., Marín Pagán, C., & Alcaraz Ramón, P. E. (2019). Effects of high
intensity circuit training frequency on isokinetic strength and body composition in
untrained subjects. Revista de Ciencias de La Actividad Física y Del Deporte de La
Universidad Católica de San Antonio, 14(41), 125-138.
https://dialnet.unirioja.es/descarga/articulo/7035800.pdf%0Ahttps://dialnet.unirioja.es/
servl et/extart?codigo=7035800

American College of Sports Medicine. Standing: the recommended amount and quality of exercise to develop and maintain cardiorespiratory and muscular fitness and flexibility in healthy adults. Sports Exercise Med Sci. 1998; 30 (6): 975-91.

Corralo, D S. (2020). Spirometry. Webconsults https://www.webconsultas.com/pruebas-medicas/espirometria-12115.

Clínica Universidad de Navarra (2019). Pneumonia: symptoms, diagnosis and treatment. Retrieved September 20, 2021, from https://www.cun.es/enfermedades-treatments/diseases/pneumonia.

Desai, S. V., Law, T. J., & Needham, D. M. (2011). Long-term complications of critical care. Critical Care Medicine, 39(2), 371-379. https://doi.org/10.1097/CCM.0b013e3181fd66e5.

General Directorate of Public Health and Food (2007). Physical activity and exercise in the elderly. 1-114.

Di Ruggiero, M. (2011, January 1). Declaration of Helsinki, bioethical principles and values at stake in medical research with human beings. Revista Colombiana de Bioética. https://revistas.unbosque.edu.co/index.php/RCB/article/view/821

Dorca, J., Bello, S., Blanquer, J., De Celis, R., Molinos, L., Torres, A., Verano, A., & Zalacain, R. (1997). Diagnosis and treatment of community-acquired pneumonia. Archivos de Bronconeumologia, 33(5), 240-246. https://doi.org/10.1016/S0300-2896(15)30614-1.

Garc, M., & Mart, B. D. (2015). Health Survey SF-36 : Validation in Three Cultural Contexts of Mexico Health Survey SF-36 : Validation in Three Cultural Contexts of Mexico Abstract. 3(871), 5-16.

García-río, F., Calle, M., Burgos, F., Casan, P., Galdiz, J. B., Giner, J., González-mangado, N., Ortega, F., & Puente, L. (2013). Spirometry. 49(9), 388-401.

Gagnon, D. D. D., Dorman, S., Ritchie, S., Mutt, S. J., Stenback, V., Walkowiak, J., & Herzig, K. H. (2019). Multi-Day Prolonged Low- to Moderate-Intensity Endurance Exercise Mimics 10(September), 1-12. https://doi.org/10.3389/fphys.2019.01123.

Garber, C. E., Blissmer, B., Deschenes, M. R., Franklin, B. A., Lamonte, M. J., Lee, I. M., Nieman, D. C., & Swain, D. P. (2011). Quantity and quality of exercise for developing and maintaining cardiorespiratory, musculoskeletal, and neuromotor fitness in apparently healthy adults: Guidance for prescribing exercise. Medicine and Science in Sports and Exercise, 43(7), 1334-1359. https://doi.org/10.1249/MSS.0b013e318213fefb

Ghodge, S., Tilaye, P., Deshpande, S., Nerkar, S., Kothary, K., Manwadkar, S., Physiotherapy, F. De, & Somaiya, K. J. (2020). Effect of pulmonary telerehabilitation on Functional capacity in COVID survivors ; An initial Evidence. 10, 123-129.

Gochicoa-Rangel L, Mora-Romero U, Guerrero-Zúñiga S, et al. Six-minute walk test: recommendations and procedures. Neumol Cir Thorax. 2019;78(Suppl: 2):164- 172. doi:10.35366/NTS192J.

Golden, C. J. (2005). Stroop test of colors and words. In TEA Ediciones.

Gonçalves, C. A. M., Dantas, P. M. S., dos Santos, I. K., Dantas, M., da Silva, D. C. P., Cabral, B. G. de A. T., Guerra, R. O., & Júnior, G. B. C. (2020). Effect of Acute and Chronic Aerobic Exercise on Immunological Markers: A Systematic Review. Frontiers in Physiology, 10(January), 1-11. https://doi.org/10.3389/fphys.2019.01602. https://doi.org/10.3389/fphys.2019.01602

Graham, B. L., Steenbruggen, I., Miller, M. R., Barjaktarevic, I. Z., Cooper, B. G., Hall, G. L., Hallstrand, T. S., Kaminsky, D. A., Mccarthy, K., Mccormack, M. C., Oropez, C. E., Rosenfeld, M., Stanojevic, S., Swanney, M. P., & Thompson, B. R. (2019). American Thoracic Society and European Respiratory Society Technical Statement. 200(8). https://doi.org/10.1164/rccm.201908-1590ST

Guo, Y., Cao, Q., Hong, Z., Tan, Y., Chen, S., Jin, H., Tan, K., Wang, D., & Yan, Y. (2020). The origin , transmission and clinical therapies on coronavirus disease 2019 (COVID-19) outbreak - an update on the status. 1-10.

Harvey, P. D., & Mohs, R. C. (2001). Memory Changes with Aging and Dementia. In functional neurobiology of aging. academic press. https://doi.org/10.1016/B978-0-12-351830-9.50007-x

Hoffman, L. A. (2007). Mobility Interventions to Improve Outcomes in Patients Undergoing Prolonged Mechanical Ventilation: A Review of the Literature.

Huang, & Zhao, N. (2020). Generalized anxiety disorder, depressive symptoms and sleep quality during COVID-19 outbreak in China: a web-based cross-sectional survey. Psychiatry Research, 288(April), 112954. https://doi.org/10.1016/j.psychres.2020.112954.

Javier, F., Gutiérrez, Á., Neumología, S. De, Reina, H., & Córdoba, S. (n.d.). Asociación de Neumólogos del Sur | Consensus document on Spirometry in Andalusia. Neumosur. http://www.neumosur.net/files/consenso_ESPIROMETRIA.pdf

Lau, H. M. C., Ng, G. Y. F., Jones, A. Y. M., Lee, E. W. C., Siu, E. H. K., & Hui, D. S. C. (2005). A randomised controlled trial of the effectiveness of an exercise training program in patients recovering from severe acute respiratory syndrome. Australian Journal of Physiotherapy, 51(4), 213-219. https://doi.org/10.1016/S0004-9514(05)70002-7

Lederer, D. J., Arcasoy, S. M., Wilt, J. S., D'Ovidio, F., Sonett, J. R., & Kawut, S. M. (2006). Six-minute-walk distance predicts waiting list survival in idiopathic pulmonary fibrosis. American Journal of Respiratory and Critical Care Medicine, 174(6), 659-664. https://doi.org/10.1164/rccm.200604-5200C.

Liu, K., Chen, Y., Wu, D., Lin, R., Wang, Z., & Pan, L. (2020). Effects of progressive muscle relaxation on anxiety and sleep quality in patients with COVID-19. Complementary Therapies in Clinical Practice, 39, 101132. https://doi.org/10.1016/j.ctcp.2020.101132. https://doi.org/10.1016/j.ctcp.2020.101132

Lj, G., Mpw, G., Ts, W., & Group, E. (2015). recovery from critical illness (Review). 6. https://doi.org/10.1002/14651858.CD008632.pub2.www.cochranelibrary.com

Martínez Vernaza, S., Soto Chávez, M. J., Mckinley, E., & Gualtero Trujillo, S. (2018). Community-acquired pneumonia: a narrative review. Universitas Médica, 59(4), 1-10. https://doi.org/10.11144/javeriana.umed59-4.neum. https://doi.org/10.11144/javeriana.umed59-4.neum

Mccormack, P., Burnham, P., & Southern, K. W. (2017). Autogenic drainage for airway clearance in cystic fibrosis. Cochrane Database of Systematic Reviews, 2017(10). https://doi.org/10.1002/14651858.CD009595.pub2. https://doi.org/10.1002/14651858.CD009595.pub2

Mcllwaine, M., Bradley, J., Elborn, J. S., & Moran, F. (2017). Personalising airway clearance in chronic lung disease. European Respiratory Review, 26(143). https://doi.org/10.1183/16000617.0086-2016.

Ministry of Health, Equality and Social Affairs (2021). Coronavirus Scientific-Technical Information. Centro de Coordinación de Alertas y Emergencias Sanitarias., 1, 73.

Miyamoto, S., Nagaya, N., Satoh, T., Kyotani, S., Sakamaki, F., Fujita, M., Nakanishi, N., & Miyatake, K. (2000). Clinical correlates and prognostic significance of six-minute walk test in patients with primary pulmonary hypertension: Comparison with cardiopulmonary exercise testing. American Journal of Respiratory and Critical Care Medicine, 161(2 I), 487-492. https://doi.org/10.1164/ajrccm.161.2.9906015.

Mohamed, A. A., & Alawna, M. (2020). Role of increasing the aerobic capacity on improving the function of immune and respiratory systems in patients with coronavirus (COVID-19): A review. Diabetes and Metabolic Syndrome: Clinical Research and Reviews, 14(4), 489496. https://doi.org/10.1016/j.dsx.2020.04.038. https://doi.org/10.1016/j.dsx.2020.04.038

Nabkasorn, C., Miyai, N., Sootmongkol, A., Junprasert, S., Yamamoto, H., Arita, M., & Miyashita, K. (2006). Effects of physical exercise on depression, neuroendocrine stress hormones and physiological fitness in adolescent females with depressive symptoms. European Journal of Public Health, 16(2), 179-184. https://doi.org/10.1093/eurpub/cki159

Nelson, M. E., Rejeski, W. J., Blair, S. N., Duncan, P. W., Judge, J. O., King, A. C., Macera, C. A., & Castaneda-Sceppa, C. (2007). Physical activity and public health in older adults: Recommendation from the American College of Sports Medicine and the American Heart Association. Circulation, 116(9), 1094-1105.

https://doi.org/10.1161/CIRCULATIONAHA.107.185650

WHO. (2020). Clinical management of COVID-19. World Health Organization, 5, 1-68. https://apps.who.int/iris/bitstream/handle/10665/332638/WHO-2019-nCoV-clinical-2 020.5- spa.pdf?sequence=1&isAllowed=y

WHO (2020) WHO Guidelines on Physical Activity and Sedentary Habits. Available at https://www.who.int/es/publications/i/item/9789240014886

Pal, M., Berhanu, G., Desalegn, C., & Kandi, V. (2020). Severe Acute Respiratory Syndrome Coronavirus-2 (SARS-CoV-2): An Update. 2(3). https://doi.org/10.7759/cureus.7423

Paneroni, M., Simonelli, C., Saleri, M., Bertacchini, L., Venturelli, M., Troosters, T., Ambrosino, N., & Vitacca, M. (2021). Muscle Strength and Physical Performance in Patients without Previous Disabilities Recovering from COVID-19 Pneumonia. American Journal of Physical Medicine and Rehabilitation, 100(2), 105-109. https://doi.org/10.1097/PHM.0000000000001641.

Park, W. B., Jun, K. Il, Kim, G., Choi, J. P., Rhee, J. Y., Cheon, S., Lee, C. H., Park, J. S., Kim, Y., Joh, J. S., Chin, B. S. S., Choe, P. G., Bang, J. H., Park, S. W., Kim, N. J., Lim, D. G., Kim, Y. S., Oh, M. don, & Shin, H. S. (2018). Correlation between pneumonia severity and pulmonary complications in Middle East respiratory syndrome. Journal of Korean Medical Science, 33(24), 1-5. https://doi.org/10.3346/jkms.2018.33.e169.

Pfeifer, M. (2020). COVID-19-Pneumonie. 793-803. https://doi.org/10.1007/s00108-020-00854-5

Properties, P. (2010). Mini-Mental State Examination MMSE - Mini-Mental State Examination Memory Changes with Aging and De- mentia Neuropsychological Testing.

Rapela, L., & Capodarco, G. (2021). Pulmonary rehabilitation in a patient hospitalized for hypoxemia post COVID-19. Acta Colombiana de Cuidado Intensivo, xxxx, 1-4. https://doi.org/10.1016/j.acci.2021.03.001

Rodríguez, M. Á., Crespo, I., & Olmedillas, H. (2020). Exercising in times of COVID-19: what do experts recommend doing within four walls? Revista Española de Cardiología, 73(7), 527-529. https://doi.org/10.1016/j.recesp.2020.04.002.

Rivero-Yeverino, D. (2019). Spirometry: Basic concepts. Revista Alergia Mexico, 66(1),
76-84. https://doi.org/10.29262/ram.v66i1.536

Rilki R., Jones J (1998) The Reliability and Validity of a 6-Minute Walk Test as a Measure of Physical
Endurance in Older Adults. Journal of Aging and Physical Activity 6(4): 363-375.
https://www.researchgate.net/publication/283837801_The_Reliability_and_Validity_of_a_6-
Minute_Walk_Test_as_a_Measure_of_Physical_Endurance_in_Older_Adults.

Saldías P, F., & Díaz P, O. (2012). Efficacy and safety of respiratory physiotherapy in adult
patients with community-acquired pneumonia. Revista Chilena de Enfermedades
Respiratorias, 28(3), 189-198. https://doi.org/10.4067/s0717- 73482012000300004.

Simioni, C., Zauli, G., Martelli, A. M., Vitale, M., Gonelli, A., & Neri, L. M. (2018).
Oncotarget-09-17181.Pdf. Oxidative Stress: Role of Physical Exercise and Antioxidant.

Nutraceuticals in Adulthood and Aging, 9(24), 17181-17198.

Strassmann, A., Steurer-Stey, C., Lana, K. D., Zoller, M., Turk, A. J., Suter, P., & Puhan, M.
A. (2013). Population-based reference values for the 1-min sit-to-stand test.
International Journal of Public Health, 58(6), 949-953.
https://doi.org/10.1007/s00038-013-0504-z.

Tirapegui S., F., Díaz P., O., & Saldías P., F. (2018). Use of systemic corticosteroids in adult
patients hospitalized for community-acquired pneumonia. Revista Chilena de
Enfermedades Respiratorias, 34(4), 236-248. https://doi.org/10.4067/s0717-
73482018000400236

Vaquero-cristobal, R., González-moro, I. M., Alacid, F., & Simón, R. (2015). Spanish
Journal of Geriatrics and Gerontology as a function of body mass index in active older
women. 48(4), 171-176.

Vega Padilla, J. D., & Barón Muñoz, E. A. (2017). Exacerbation of chronic obstructive
pulmonary disease. Medicina General y de Familia, 6(4), 167-171.
https://doi.org/10.24038/mgyf.2017.032

Vilagut, G., Ferrer, M., Rajmil, L., Rebollo, P., Permanyer-Miralda, G., Quintana, J. M.,

Santed, R., Valderas, J. M., Ribera, A., Domingo-Salvany, A., & Alonso, J. (2005). The Spanish version of the Short Form 36 Health Survey: a decade of experience and new developments. Gaceta Sanitaria / S.E.S.S.P.A.S, 19(2), 135-150. https://doi.org/10.1157/13074369

Wang, T. J., Chau, B., Lui, M., Lam, G. T., Lin, N., & Humbert, S. (2020). Physical medicine and rehabilitation and pulmonary rehabilitation for COVID-19. American Journal of Physical Medicine and Rehabilitation, 99(9), 769-774. https://doi.org/10.1097/PHM.0000000000001505.

Yurainys, A., Candelaria, B., Angie, C., Anyi, C., Liceth, G., Machado, A., Yulieth, M., Martinez, M., Orenis, U., Fabiana, P., Pineda, R., Ramirez, Y., Rodelo, M., Villegas, V., & Palacio, I. (2015). Physiotherapeutic approach of a patient with community-acquired pneumonia: a case study. Rev. Salud Mov., 7(1), 19-32.

Zhao, H. M., Xie, Y. X., & Wang, C. (2020). Recommendations for respiratory rehabilitation in adults with coronavirus disease 2019. Chinese Medical Journal, 133(13), 1595-1602.

https://doi.org/10.1097/CM9.0000000000000848

Zhou, P., Yang, X., Wang, X., Hu, B., Zhang, L., Zhang, W., Guo, H., Jiang, R., Liu, M., Chen, Y., Shen, X., Wang, X., Zhan, F., Wang, Y., Xiao, G., & Shi, Z. (2020). A pneumonia outbreak associated with a new coronavirus of probable bat origin. Nature, 579(March). https://doi.org/10.1038/s41586-020-2012-7

11. Anexos

Anexo A. Consentimiento Informado

Consentimiento Informado para participar Voluntariamente en una

investigación

Estimado Sr ____

Usted ha sido invitado a participar en el estudio titulado, **"Efectos de un programa de ejercicio aeróbico combinado con terapia respiratoria sobre la condición física, calidad de vida relacionada con la salud y funciones ejecutivas en un sobreviviente de neumonía por SARS-CoV-2"** realizada por, Alex Chacón Sevilla, Estudiante del Máster Universitario en Actividad Física y Calidad de Vida en personas adultas y mayores, de la Universidad de Sevilla, España.

El objetivo de esta investigación es, Determinar los efectos de un Programa de Ejercicio Aeróbico moderado combinado con Terapia Respiratoria, para mejorar la capacidad cardiopulmonar, la fuerza muscular, funciones ejecutivas y calidad vida relacionada con la salud, en un sobreviviente de neumonía atípica bilateral inducida por SARS-CoV-2, tras su alta hospitalaria.

En este estudio nos ayudará a comprender más sobre, como el ejercicio físico aeróbico puede tener un efecto sobre las capacidades cardiopulmonares y la fuerza muscular. Los resultados de esta investigación podrían mejorar la condición física de los pacientes que hoy están padeciendo el mismo problema de salud al suyo.

Su participación es totalmente voluntaria y puede tomarse el tiempo que requiera para decidir participar. Durante todo el estudio, el personal que desarrolla el proyecto, está a su disposición para aclarar cualquier duda o inquietud que usted tenga.

Aunque haya decidido participar, usted puede retirarse del estudio en cualquier momento, sin explicación. Su atención médica presente y futura no cambiará de ninguna manera, si usted decide no participar.

La participación consistirá en un estudio de caso. Usted será la única persona que participará en dicha investigación. El procedimiento se realizará en primer lugar en su domicilio y en segundo lugar en el Gimnasio de la ciudad, y en tercer lugar en los espacios abiertos de su comunidad. Dicho programa lo llevara a cabo el investigador a cargo y tiene una duración de 8 semanas con una frecuencia de 3 días semanales.

Los datos obtenidos serán de carácter confidencial, se guardará el anonimato en el ordenador del investigador, la identidad de su persona estará disponible sólo para el personal del proyecto y se mantendrá completamente privado. Los datos estarán a cargo del investigador responsable y de su tutor de investigación y para el posterior desarrollo de informes y publicaciones dentro de revistas científicas. Todos los nuevos resultados significativos desarrollados durante el curso de la investigación, le serán entregados a Usted. Además, se entregará un informe con los resultados generales sin identificar su nombre.

Si Usted no desea participar no implicará sanción. Usted tiene el derecho a negarse a responder a preguntas concretas, también puede optar por retirarse de este estudio en cualquier momento y la información que hemos recogido será descartada del estudio y eliminada.

También para esta investigación existen riesgos que son particulares de la práctica del ejercicio físico (Fatiga muscular, lesiones, caídas, cansancio). Si así lo desea, puede dejar de participar en las actividades que considere un riesgo para su salud, sin que signifique sanción para Usted. De participar de todo el estudio los beneficios directos serán; Su recuperación física, enfermedad, condición o síntomas secundarios, sin embargo, no existen garantías que ello ocurra, además otro beneficio es mejorar su capacidad cardiopulmonar y la fuerza muscular y la posibilidad de ayudar a desarrollar programas de intervención para personas en su misma situación de salud. No se contemplan ningún otro tipo de beneficios.

Las informaciones recolectadas no serán usadas para ningún otro propósito, además de los señalados anteriormente, sin su autorización previa y por escrito.

Por último, informarle que para esta investigación se tomaran en cuenta todas las medidas de seguridad ante el contagio de la COVID-19 (uso de mascarilla, lavado de manos con gel hidroalcohólico o con agua y jabón, desinfección de los instrumentos utilizados, distancia de seguridad, entre otras).

Cualquier pregunta que Usted desee hacer durante el proceso de investigación podrá contactar con el responsable de dicho estudio; Alex Chacón Sevilla, Estudiante del Máster Universitario en Actividad Física y Calidad de Vida de Personas Adultas y Mayores de la Universidad de Sevilla.

Correo electrónico: jose88danh@gmail.com, en horario de 09:00 a 20:00 horas, de lunes a sábados. **Agradezco desde ya su colaboración DNI/NIE Participante Firma**

Annex B

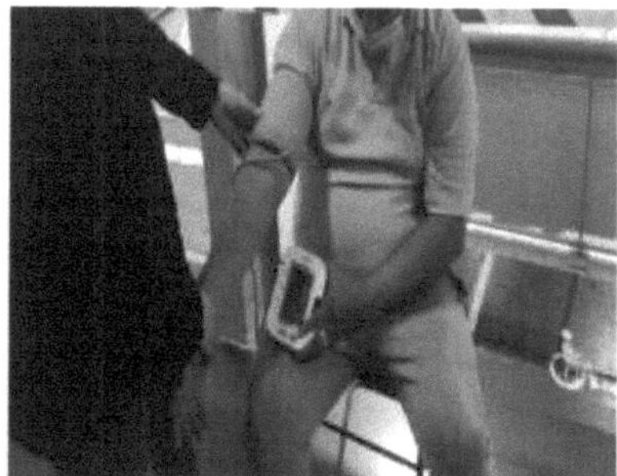

Figure B 1. Note: Blood pressure and Sat0$_2$ before the 6-minute walk test 6.

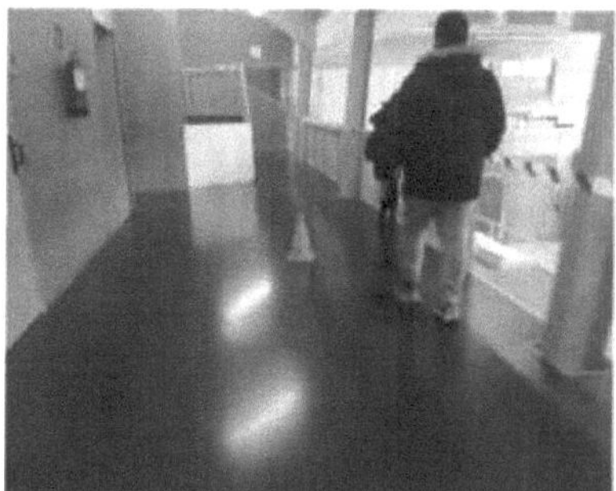

Figure B 2 Note: Performance of the 6 min test, the cones are distance indicators.

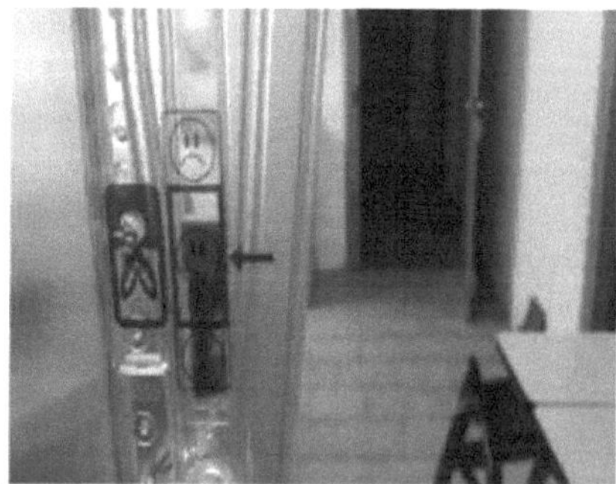

Figure B 3. Note: Incentive spirometer used for respiratory therapy.

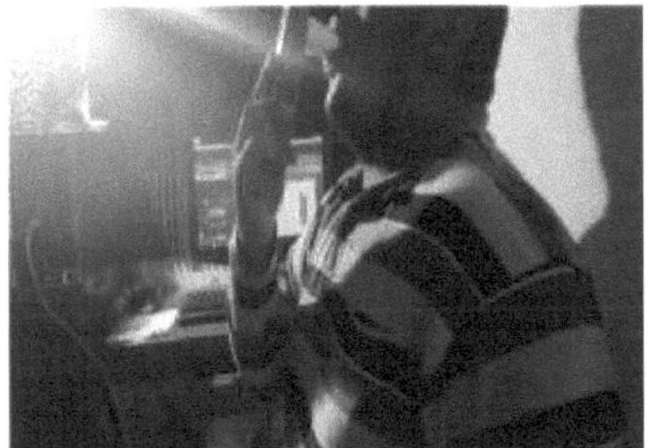

Figure B 4. Note: Performance of forced spirometry.

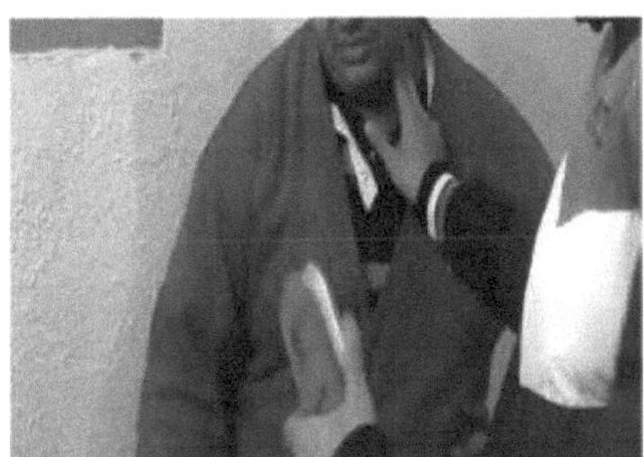

Figure B 5. Note: Manual control of HR.

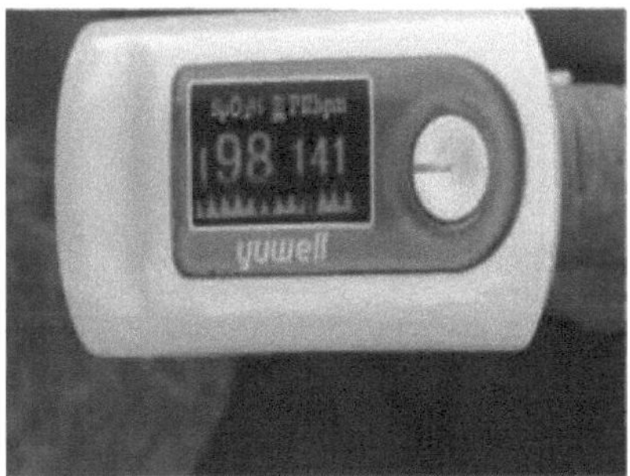

Figure B 6. Note: Pulse oximeter, for monitoring of Sat02 and HR.

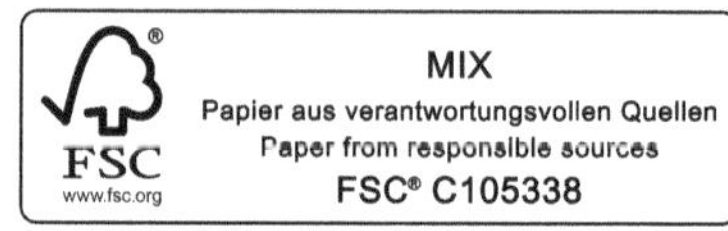

Printed by Books on Demand GmbH, Norderstedt / Germany